6 Proven Eating Habits to Shed Unwanted Pounds Forever

(And the Top Ten Reasons Why People Fail to Lose Weight)

RON KNESS

Contents

Introduction

One reason most people fall off the weight loss wagon after making heart-felt and sincere commitments is that the new habits they're trying to form are stressful and set up to make them fail.

But my book - **6 Proven Eating Habits to Shed Unwanted Pounds Forever** - is different; it charts a weight loss plan that can help you make lifetime changes that will help you maintain your ideal weight. It's the little habits which can make a huge difference and the advice contained in this book will be both obvious and eye opening.

Within these pages, you'll learn how distractions can cause mindless eating and pack on the calories without you even realizing it. Portion control is also a big factor in achieving your weight loss goals – even the celebrities lose unwanted pounds by watching their portions.

How you prepare your food is a good indicator of how many calories you're going to consume. You know that baking is healthier and doles out less calories than deep frying – but you'll also learn some other ways to enjoy high-calorie old family recipes with half the calorie count.

Now is the time to try new foods and expand your culinary knowledge to other lands. Many diet plans – such as Mediterranean – offer tasty meals using ingredients you may have never used before.

You'll learn how to transform boring recipes using these amazing ingredients that are much healthier and lower in calories. Mindful eating can work when all else fails. This plan allows you to eat what you desire, but also teaches you to recognize the triggers telling you when you've had enough to eat.

Hunger cues are all-important if you have a tendency to eat after you're full just because it tastes good or you're eating based on emotions. Finally, you'll be happy to learn some ways you can still enjoy "fast food" without feeling guilty afterward.

Guilt is a horrible word for dieters. It signifies failure. But, with the new eating habits in my book, you can get rid of the word "guilt" and begin to live life with restored health and vigor and build good habits a little bit at a time.

Most bad habits need to be replaced with good and useful ones or you revert back to the old habits. This book will provide the tools you need to replace the old habits that are adding fat to your body and harming your health by showing you ways to look at and enjoy food at its very best.

You'll soon come to enjoy the new habits acquired and the results you realize will seem like they were easier to achieve than what you may have seen in the past.

You'll be savoring your food so much more -- and the result will be losing weight and being able to maintain it throughout your life.

But before we delve into these proven eating habits, let's first talk about the top ten reasons why people fail to lose weight.

Top 10 Reasons Why People Fail to Lose Weight

Too many people set out to lose weight and end up failing or giving up. The good news is that being prepared and understanding *why* people fail can help prevent you making the same mistakes. Go through this list, see if any of them sound like something you've done (or not done) and discover how you can overcome these failures so you can start using our proven tips to lose the weight and keep it off forever.

#10 Doing a fad diet

Fad diets don't work. That's the main reason they get coined with the term "fad." They are here today and gone tomorrow. Only eating plans that have stood the test of time lose the phrase "fad diet" and become popular and well known. Atkins and South Beach that are two that have stood the test of time and turned into healthy eating plans. Many doctors and nutritionist are finally coming on board with these two diets.

Following the latest diet craze in the newest edition of some women's magazine is generally not a diet or eating plan you will stick to in the long run. To ensure you have life-long results, you need to make life-long sustainable changes in your eating habits.

#9 Eating too few calories

You know you need to cut calories to lose weight, but restricting your caloric intake too severely will not only have adverse effects on your body, this plan will back fire. A calorie is a unit of fuel. Your body needs fuel to function.

When you restrict your daily calorie intake too far below what you need, the body will think it's going into starvation mode and will start taking nutrients from the muscles. You need those muscles. A better approach is to eat the recommended daily calorie allowance for your size and weight loss goals and start adding some muscle building exercises.

Muscles burn fat so adding more muscle will keep your metabolism and the fat burning process going. You may notice a slight increase in weight at first, but keep it up. Before long you'll notice the pounds of fat coming off because the muscles are using that fat as energy/fuel.

#8 Going too long between meals

Waiting too long to eat can have negative effects in your weight loss process too. The body's metabolism keeps at a good pace as long as it has something to work with. When you skip meals or wait too long the eat, it will slow down your metabolism, thus slowing down the fat burning process as well. It's best to eat several small meals per day, plus have several snacks in between meals. Make sure these are healthy snacks, but eating every few hours will keep your metabolism stoked and ready to go.

#7 Unrealistic weight loss goals

Setting unrealistic weight loss goals, like expecting to lose ten pounds in one week is another cause of failure. If you don't lose those ten pounds you'll soon give up trying. A better goal is one pound per week. That doesn't sound like much, but over the course of a several weeks or even months it will add up. You didn't put on those extra pounds in a few days, you can't expect to lose them in a few days either. In fact, it may take longer to lose them than it did to gain them.

#6 Failing to organize and plan ahead

Not planning ahead and being organized with your weight loss plans is another cause of failure. If you don't have a plan or a goal to reach, how do you expect to get there? Having a plan means you know when to add an exercise or change up your routine, how many days per week you plan to workout, or even there will be days you need to watch your calories more closely because of a special occasion.

#5 Failing to stock up on the right foods

If you don't have healthy foods and snacks in your home, you're more likely to grab some junk food when you get hungry. You have to keep good foods on hand so they are available to you at all times. Keep fresh fruits and vegetables well stocked so you can grab those instead of cookies or crackers the next time you want a snack. Go ahead and chop some up into bite-sized pieces and keep them in storage containers so you can grab them quickly.

This is especially helpful if you've gone too long without eating and need something quick.

#4 Failing to get rid of temptations

If you keep bad foods around, like chips, cookies, cake or crackers you're more likely to grab those for a quick fix when you get hungry. The old saying, "Out of sight, out of mind," is especially true of food. If you're craving something and it's in your home, chances are you will grab it instead of the fruit or other healthy snacks. Make sure you clean out your pantry before trying a new weight loss plan.

#3 Not exercising

It doesn't matter how much you cut your calories, you'll get faster results if you exercise. There are many fad diets that claim you can lose weight without exercise, but the truth is the body was designed to move. You don't have to jump into a full-blown fitness guru mode, but you do need to start getting more daily activity into your routine. You can start by walking or doing a light aerobics training a few times each week. It doesn't have to be complicated. Simply start getting out and moving more so you speed up the fat burning process and get your metabolism into a higher gear.

#2 Not having a plan

This is similar to the one above. If you don't have a plan made out for your weight loss journey you won't have guidelines to stick to. It's much easier to give up if you don't have something written down on your calendar to remind you to get out and exercise or when to increase your exercise. Also, if you plan to introduce new foods into your eating plan, you need some kind of guide to go by. You may want to add one food per week or one every other week. When you have this written down you don't have to question when or which food it is, you simply look at your plan.

#1 Failing to start

The number one reason that people don't reach weight loss success is that they simply don't start. They keep talking about it, maybe even keep planning it, but until they take action and start working those plans, nothing will happen.

You don't have to start off with starving yourself. You just need to start. You can start by cutting out some junk foods and replacing them with healthier snacks. Start walking 2 or 3 days per week until you can work up to more.

The key to success with anything is to start the program. Sticking to it may be hard, but until you start you will not get anywhere.

Don't set yourself up to fail at losing weight. Plan ahead, have healthy, low-fat food at hand, eat regularly and get enough calories so you don't slow down your metabolism, and do the exercise. Now onto the good habits to achieve weight loss.

Chapter 1: Get Rid of Distractions

It's been the norm for quite some time now to eat meals and snack in front of the television. Some of our favorite sitcoms – not to mention the news – come on at dinner time and there was no way to record and watch them later until the advent of DVRs.

This habit has wrecked eating habits and made family dinners a thing of the past for most Americans. In Europe and Asia, people still sit down as a family for meals, which is precisely why those countries have less obesity than America.

Working on the computer while you eat is also a way to consume mindless calories and not even be aware of the delicious food you're eating. Shoving pizza in your mouth as you play a fast-paced game doesn't do much for your digestion either.

Halting the habit of mindless eating can cut calories and help you enjoy your food more – plus, make you healthier because you eat slower and in a place of serenity rather than a place that breeds chaos.

Distractions Keep You from Enjoying Your Food

You're missing a lot when you choose to eat your meals in front of the television or engage in other distractions. You don't really savor the special textures, flavors or aromas of a well thought-out meal, nor do you give your body a chance to communicate with your brain, telling you when you've had enough.

We've all salivated over the aroma of a savory roast in the crock pot, cookies or bread baking in the oven or fresh coffee, bacon and eggs in the early morning. There's a theory that eating by following your senses can help you lose weight.

When you focus on the texture, taste, aroma, sight and touch of food, you're less likely to overeat. But, being able to focus on the meals you're eating means that you must get rid of the distractions that are taking away the power of those senses and causing you to engage in mindless eating habits.

Presentation (sight) is very important in the process of enjoying your food. A roasted chicken, cut up and plopped on a platter is much less appetizing than the same chicken placed on a platter with roasted potatoes, onions and carrots surrounding it – and perhaps a sprig or two of parsley for a pop of color.

Eating by using your senses is the missing ingredient in most meals today. Weight loss experts call it a "sensory disregard," and consider it a portent of overeating and eventual obesity.

This means that if you're not enjoying each meal through your senses, you're likely going to keep eating until you're way over the food intake for one meal.

Some tricks to enjoy your food even more by paying attention to your sense include drizzling extra virgin olive oil over fresh salad greens or over warm, whole-grain bread.

Pay close attention to your table setting and be sure everything is colorful and serene. Also, savor each bite for taste and texture to determine whether it's sweet, salty, bitter or another taste.

Feeding your senses requires you to seek and develop a new relationship with food. This new habit can transform how you think about meals and drastically cut your calories to help you lose weight.

How Distractions Cause Weight Gain

Distractions cause your body to store more fat than it should because it doesn't work at its peak efficiency when you're distracted. Nutrients aren't processed as effectively as they should be and your body is tricked into believing that you need more calories to produce energy.

Your brain is concentrating on the distraction rather than the meal and forgets to send the message to your stomach to quit eating – you've had enough. The distraction causes you to eat much more than it needs at the moment and ends up storing it as – fat.

Eventually, you'll suffer the domino effect that distractions cause by having a stomach that's too large so it can take on the extra food that's being consumed. You may not feel full anymore, even after eating a large, high calorie meal.

So, you go back to the kitchen for snacks to munch on in the front of the television or computer. More mindless eating. To stop this endless cycle of eating while being distracted, you've got to realize what is distracting you.

If it's the television, the answer is simple. Turn it off, eat in another room and record the programs for another time, when you're not eating. Have you noticed how you eat when you're engrossed in a favorite program or good movie?

If you're in the theater, you're likely shoving popcorn or Junior Mints into your mouth at an astounding rate. You might as well be eating the box as what's in it for all the satisfaction you're getting.

Many of us eat at the table, but bring a magazine, newspaper or book to the table to "have something to do" while eating. Kids now bring cell phones to the table and text their friends while at the meal table.

Even music may be a distraction if it's played to the tune of a fast beat because it makes you want to eat faster. Some restaurants purposely play an upbeat tempo in the background.

Although you may not be aware of the actual music, the beat causes you to eat faster and leave earlier so other customers can take your place. No matter what distractions you're prone to at mealtimes, your brain doesn't register that you have reached maximum capacity in your stomach and you just keep eating.

Techniques for Focusing on the Meal

Allowing distractions during meals is a bad habit that can be broken with some forethought and planning. After you learn these techniques and put them into practice, you'll be surprised at how much less you're eating and how much better and more satisfied you feel.

Always sit at a nicely set table, free from books, gadgets and phones and away from the television, computer or any other thing that may constitute a distraction. Rather than putting bowls and platters on the table, fill your plate from the stove or countertop with smaller portions than you're used to.

One technique that mindful eating enthusiasts advocate is to put less food on your fork or spoon. This one little trick will give you more bang for the buck at your meals by providing more bites, but less food – and calories.

After each bite, put down your knife and fork and remove your hands from the table. Chew your food slowly and savor the flavors, textures and aromas. This serves to help you enjoy your food so much more and become satisfied with less.

Don't pick up your knife and fork again until you've chewed and swallowed the last bite you put in your mouth. No matter how much food is left on the plate – stop when you feel full and satisfied.

The fact that you're eating slower gives your brain time to register the contents of your stomach and stops you from wanting more when you're full. Your digestive system will become more efficient in channeling your nutrients to the proper areas and getting rid of the intake of fat that you don't need rather than storing it.

Your metabolism also works much more efficiently and will keep working even after the meal to burn extra calories rather than getting bogged down with an overload that makes it sluggish and ineffective.

It's been proven that a colorful plate of food is likely filled with the nutrition you need for optimum health. Be sure the color green is represented in salads or healthy greens. Orange carrots and brown, multi-grain bread also add to the color scheme of a healthy meal.

Developing mindful eating habits should also steer you clear of processed foods and unhealthy items such as foods fried in animal fat and snacks laden with sugar and chemicals.

Next time you plan a meal, incorporate some of the above methods. It may take a while, but you'll soon find that you're enjoying the new eating habits and are gaining a new respect for food and how it should be presented – and eaten.

Distractions Discourage Mindful Eating

There is a concept derived from the Buddhist belief of being totally aware of what is happening around you and within your body at every waking moment. This concept is believed to reduce stress and help alleviate chronic health problems such as digestive and blood pressure ailments.

The mindful eating concept is derived from this Buddhist belief and encourages people to keep from eating too much food and to stay away from processed and unhealthy foods.

When you're aware of what you're eating – and the senses are completely involved, you're more thoughtful about how much you eat. It's a way of helping the brain communicate with the gut by sending signals that are not ignored because you're distracted by something else while you're eating.

The hormones involved in the digestion process connects the nervous system to the stomach and may take up to 20 minutes for the brain to get the signal that it's satisfied and ready to quit eating.

If you eat too quickly (while watching television or reading a book), you'll likely not give the connection enough time to get and respond to the signals.

Mindful eating has also been studied as a strategy for binge-eaters and others with eating disorders which lead to obesity.

In a recent study involving 150 binge-eaters, it was concluded that mindfulness-based therapy helped the control group enjoy their food more and eat less. As with any new way of eating, begin the mindful eating process gradually.

Start with a meal once a week in which you consume it in a slower, more fixed manner rather than a helter-skelter approach in front of the television, at your desk or computer. Before you begin to consume your meal, set the kitchen timer for 20 minutes and eat with your non-dominant hand (if you're right handed, hold the fork in your left hand to eat).

Chopsticks will also slow down the eating process if you're not proficient at using them. Also, eat in silence for five minutes, thinking always about the food you're consuming – the color, texture, aroma and other factors such as bitter, salty or sweet.

Think of how the food was grown and about the sunshine and rain that helped it along. Take very small bites and chew each one well. Soon, this method will add a new dimension to your enjoyment of eating.

You'll be savoring the food rather than mindlessly scarfing it down. Remember, no distractions = less food consumption.

Chapter 2: Change the Way You Serve Yourself

It sounds so simple, doesn't it? If you don't serve yourself large and calorie-laden portions, you're bound to lose weight. But our society doesn't run on tiny portions. Even the dishes we use now are twice as large as those our grandparents ate from.

As a society, we're consuming more food than ever – and exercising less. As a result, we've become a society of obese people who yo-yo back and forth on diet and exercise plans which render our bodies and minds confused and make losing weight even more difficult.

Changing the way you serve yourself is part of the mindful eating concept that advocates you being aware of everything you put in your mouth and everything around you as you're eating.

Mindful eating is a lifestyle change that you'll eventually enjoy because not only will you lose unwanted pounds – you'll become much more aware of how your body and mind work together when you eat.

Knowledge is power and with mindful eating techniques you can make a real and significant lifestyle change. There is much more to how you serve yourself than watching your portion size.

And, you may choose a small portion of something that has a much higher impact in calories than a double serving of something else.

This chapter of *6 Proven Eating Habits to Help Shed Unwanted Pounds Forever* will show you the importance of other aspects of how you serve yourself, such as color, aroma, size of dishes and a quick way to measure some foods without using a scale.

Serving Techniques for Weight Loss

Serving size is important to any weight loss plan, including mindful eating. Rather than taking the time and effort to memorize how much is in an ounce, cup and various measuring spoons, try comparing them to other items you're familiar with.

For example, a serving of pasta is roughly the size of a normal scoop of ice cream. If you're eating a single serving of a vegetable or fruit, visualize it as the size of your fist. A serving of fish, poultry or meat would fit in the palm of your hand and if you're having a snack of pretzels, use a handful as your measuring device.

One serving of a bagel is about the size of a hockey puck and the radius of a CD should be used for one serving of pancakes. The point is that you don't have to be exact when doling out food servings – a good estimate should get you to where you need to be.

If you have trouble discerning a cup versus a cup and a half of rice, put the cooked rice in a measuring cup and then empty it onto the plate for a while until you get used to the how the portion looks.

After you've eaten your meal, don't go back for seconds. When you learn and practice the mindful eating techniques mentioned in Chapter 1: Get Rid of Distractions, you should feel more satisfied after the meal.

Serve yourself from the counter or stove and immediately put away all the leftovers in their proper portions – freezing them if you aren't likely to eat them right away. Out of sight – out of mind.

Always eat from the plate or bowl rather than from a carton or bag. It's easy to miscalculate portions when digging into a container. Use smaller dishes to eat from rather than the dinner plates we're more used to now.

If you're at a restaurant, prepare to receive huge portions of food. Ask for smaller portions if possible or eat what you estimate is a portion and put the remainder in a doggie bag.

It's okay to order dessert, but be sure to share or take part of it home for another time. When food shopping, be aware of food labeled as "mini-snacks" which come in small containers but carry a truckload of calories.

You'll likely eat more than you planned – especially if you're eating from the bag. If you can, shop for individual-sized servings – at least until you become more familiar with portion sizes.

Eating ice cream from the carton is a real, diet-deal-breaker. It makes you more mindful of how much you're eating to choose individual ice cream servings such as ice-cream sandwiches or ice cream bars.

For an easy route to learning portion size servings, check out the new dishes which are specially designed for helping people learn and execute new eating habits involving smaller portions for weight loss. I review a couple of different small plate options in the Product Review chapter at the end of this book.

Serving Yourself Sensibly

There are so many ways to trick yourself into being satisfied with less food. It's a known fact that portion size has increased to abominable heights. A recent study in Australia pursued the reality of our dishes and portion size to the fact we're becoming a society of obese people.

This study even analyzed plate types (cone-shaped or flat) for calorie density and compared those findings to the daily, recommended calorie allowance. The results proved that even a small increase in the size of the dishes can cause an enormous increase in consumed calories.

So, dishware size is a definite consideration when using mindful eating techniques to lose and maintain weight. Other factors besides the size of the dishware were whether a bowl or plate was chosen, how the dish was filled and how calorie-dense the food was.

Interestingly enough, the plate or bowl filling and the shape of the plate also depends on the individuals serving themselves. Some people fill up the dishes to the maximum capacity and others were more mindful of the portions.

Ambiance Is Everything

Dish size is important, but the ambiance of where you eat is essential if you're going to take full advantage of the mindful eating concept. We can't all eat in the atmosphere of Downton Abby each night, being served by butlers and servants.

But, you can take what you have and make it into a place of serenity and peace to eat your meals.

The fact is that most people now take their meals in front of the television, computer, in bed, standing up on a commuter train or in casual restaurants that serve huge portions of deep fried foods on plastic trays.

At home, meals are sometimes taken on the run like a marathon you have to finish so you can get to the next appointment or practice session. Most of the time, one family member at a time serves him or herself and disappears with a plateful of food to consume it in front of the television or while on the phone in their rooms.

Meals are seldom planned, much less served in an environment that's conducive of calm rather than chaos. Does it really matter whether we're on the run, eating in the ambiance of an elegant restaurant or in front of the television? Science says it does.

Any restaurant that goes to the trouble to put together a five-star menu is likely to go to the trouble of making the ambiance match the food. That doesn't mean white tablecloths and flowers on the table, but it should match the type of food.

For example, a barbeque restaurant may have checkered tablecloths, paper towels for napkins and lots of country music playing in the background. Chefs know that the eating experience comprises both the psychological and physiological needs and wants of the diner and the body and mind respond to the surroundings.

While you may not be able to recreate the atmosphere of a five-star restaurant at home, you can use color, candles and a warm and inviting atmosphere to make your family want to dine rather than eat on the run.

For breakfast, you may want to create a light and airy atmosphere that's conducive to eating a hearty and healthy meal before going off to school and work. Lunch can be casual if you eat at home, but be sure you don't eat in front of the television or computer. Eat at the table and eat slowly.

Also keep in mind that if you consistently eat with a book in hand or in front of the television, you're setting up cues for hunger (or it makes you think you're hungry). When you reach for a book or turn on the television, you'll likely begin to crave certain foods that you associate with that activity.

The Joy of Eating

The mindful eating concept must also incorporate a joy of eating. Meals have historically been a time to enjoy family and friends and take part in the bounty that the earth has provided.

Today, the joy of eating seems to have lost its sheen and brought down to foods we crave rather than savor. Consumed on the run or while being entertained, food has lost the original happiness and celebratory mood that it used to bring to the table.

There is a movement to get back to mindful and joyful eating and to improve the relationship that many now have with food. Rather than being seen as a path to health and energy, it's now an addiction for some and a reason to turn on television or play a computer game for others.

Mindful eating is designed to bring a new way to look at the consumption of food – as sustaining and health-motivating as well as a fun and interesting way to join family and friends for a well-thought out and tasteful meal.

Food brings joy to celebrations and each meal should be a celebration of being able to eat nutritious and tasteful food – rather than how much you can consume in a short amount of time.

How you think about the food you eat and learning to meet the various needs you have without hoarding and consuming too much food is part of the mindful eating concept. Food can be interesting and fun and the more you learn about it, the more you'll appreciate it.

You'll eat for satisfaction and to get the most nutrition as possible from what you choose to eat. You'll also learn to prepare the food for the utmost nutritional value and choose portions and dishware according to what you know is an acceptable limit.

Mindful eating is a sort of revolution of changing the way people think about food. It's full of strategies and techniques to bring joy and mindfulness to every meal you make and every bite you take.

It's not as much a diet plan as it is a way to gain power over your relationship with food. Food is treated as an ally rather than an enemy and the old habits of eating without thinking are replaced with habits that promote a complete understanding and evaluation in what and how we're eating.

It may take a while to change the old habits and you may miss sitting in front of the television while mindlessly eating a pizza, but your new lifestyle will put you much more in the present moment.

A Lifestyle Change is Necessary

If you're going to embark on a mindful eating journey, you've got to make a commitment to a drastic lifestyle change. Learning to recognize hunger cues is also important to the mindful eating journey.

When you're aware of what and how you're eating, you recognize those cues and act accordingly. From the dishes you choose to the food you purchase and the way you prepare and present it, mindful eating can't be accomplished fully without a complete lifestyle change.

You can begin small, with one meal a week, but eventually, the entire concept of mindful eating will be a choice you'll gladly make. We live in such a fast-paced society that slowing down to enjoy meals with family and loved ones may feel that you've gone back in time for a while.

You'll choose food differently, even if you're forced to choose it from a vending machine or cafeteria. Focusing your thoughts on healthy food choices will also serve to help you make good choices in other areas of your life. You may take extra time and exploration to think through every issue that comes your way.

With mindful eating, you'll make choices made on the issues of health and portions rather than immediate gratification. You won't wonder anymore where the plate of pasta went – you'll know exactly, because you'll savor every bite as you eat.

Although part of the joy of mindful eating comes from sharing meals with friends and family, be aware of how others are eating and don't try to match their speed or intensity. Others may choose huge portions, but you will know instinctively how much to dole out on your plate or bowl.

The busier you get in your life, the more you may be tempted to combine a meal or snack with a chance to watch television or get some work done. Guard against that habit, although times may occur when it's necessary.

Don't blame yourself or feel guilty if you do experience a period where you're totally unmindful of what you eat or where you eat it. Old habits die hard – or circumstances may get in the way of what you know you should be doing and what time or other problems dictate you must be doing.

After you know what's expected of your mindful eating experience, you'll know instinctively when and how to serve portions, how to make the presentation of food a delight to the senses and exactly the foods you should be eating for the maximum benefit and the most weight loss.

Chapter 3: Implement Healthier Cooking Methods

Mama's fried chicken just can't be beat, but if you ate it every day you'd have a good chance of developing heart disease, high blood pressure and any number of ailments. Decades ago, much of the population worked hard and burned off excess calories and most of the damage fried foods can cause.

Today, many of us are still eating the same type of fried foods from fast food places and right in our own homes. Mindful eating techniques include implementing healthier methods of cooking into your life, but still getting the same satisfaction and taste.

Some ways of cooking that will lighten the meal include grilling, baking, roasting, poaching, sautéing, steaming and broiling. You can also stir fry meats and veggies together in a wok and use a bit of vegetable stock, wine or a bit of olive oil for seasoning.

There are so many ways to boost flavor and cut calories in your cooking techniques that you'll soon be able to look at your old, calorie-laden recipes and immediately know which substitutions to make for health and weight loss.

Don't think you have to take gourmet cooking classes or invest in an entirely new set of cookware to prepare healthy food. Mindful cooking techniques include such simple changes such as using olive oil and vinegar on salads and adding seasonings for flavor can perk up a recipe and lighten the calorie load.

A Quick Course in Healthy Cooking Techniques

You don't have to be a chef to prepare quick and healthy meals for yourself and/or your family. Frozen and prepackaged meals sometimes contain harmful preservatives and are loaded with unnecessary calories.

If you're challenge is to develop healthier eating habits, you should know some basic techniques to cut calories, choose food high in nutrients and how to avoid excess fat – without losing flavor.

You may be familiar with some of the techniques, but others will be new and different and you'll be amazed at how little time it takes to master them and use them in your daily meal preparation.

Steaming is one method that can be used to cut calories and seal in the true flavor of whatever you're cooking. Steaming can be accomplished in several ways – using a covered metal basket (perforated) that fits above a pot of boiling water, using parchment paper or foil or make it even more convenient by investing in an electric steamer pot.

Steaming eliminates the need for oil or other fats, seals in the flavor of the food and preserves the nutritional value. Best of all, it helps keep the food moist and tender – especially fish.

Don't salt foods during the steaming process as it just evaporates – and try flavoring with lemon, garlic, fresh grated ginger, basil and onion. Broiling is another technique for healthy cooking which differs from grilling in that the heat for grilling comes from below the food and broiling requires heat from above it.

You may want to marinate meat first before broiling because it's a dry heat that can dry out the meat if not prepared correctly. Chefs prefer to broil salmon and beef over other types of meat because they are naturally oily and won't tend to dry out as easy.

Other foods that are great for broiling include Cornish game hen and veggies such as squash, onion and bell pepper. Be sure to preheat the broiler so the food will be seared when you place it under the broiler.

Turn the food at the halfway point of cooking and for a quick clean-up method, line the broiler pan with foil. Pressure cooking takes very little time and retains the vitamins and minerals of your food.

Steam also seals in the flavors of the food, eliminating the need for oils or fat. You can also season the food, but it won't need much – especially if you're making stews or soups.

Chicken, risotto, soups, stews, beans and beef are just a few of the foods that can be pressure cooked and enjoyed in a brief amount of time. The pressure cooker does all the work and you get all the benefit.

Be sure to follow the instructions on your pressure cooker for safety and the best way to cook certain foods. Pressure cookers can range from $25 to $300 and become one of the best investments in your arsenal of cooking utensils.

The ancient cooking method of stir-frying is a wonderful way to cook your meals in a hurry and enjoy amazing flavors and other benefits. When you stir-fry, you're cooking the food on very intense heat for a very short amount of time.

This requires that your food is prepared by cutting into small, exact pieces so you're sure that everything is cooked done in the same amount of time.

You'll need to constantly monitor and stir the food while cooking to be sure it doesn't stick to the pan.

You may want to invest in a wok to achieve the best method of stir-frying. A wok is a round-bottom and slope-sided pan that's specially designed to be able to move food up around the sloping sides after it's done.

There are some amazing recipes for stir-fried meals, but the best foods to use include cabbage, bell peppers, mushrooms, shrimp, chicken, tofu and broccoli. The price of woks varies a great deal – from $20 to $200 (electric).

You may use your microwave only to heat up frozen dinners or warm up leftovers, but microwaving is also a great way to quickly cook fresh foods while preserving nutrients and leaving off oils and fat.

A microwave actually steams your food. Vegetables are great for microwaving because they retain their beautiful colors as well as their vitamins and minerals. Broccoli, potatoes, carrots, fish and chicken are great candidates for microwaving.

To get the most out of your microwaving experience, be sure to cover the food so that the steam retains moisture. You can use plastic wrap, but many chefs recommend a covered casserole dishes or cover a plate of food with another plate to cook.

Use your microwave's instructions to time the food. Microwaves vary in wattage, so it may take some trial and error to get it right. Some have carousels which turn the food as it's cooking, helping it to cook evenly.

Other methods include baking, which doesn't require adding fat to the food; poaching allows food to be cooked in water or a liquid consisting of broth, wine, vinegar or a combination; braising to sear the food and cook with a small amount of liquid; roasting is a method which uses the oven to cook the food until done.

Try new methods of cooking to expand your knowledge and your culinary experience. Use your old recipes to spur your creativity and find ways to cook that you'll enjoy and that will reduce calories and provide a healthier meal for you and your family.

Using Herbs and Spices to Jazz Up Your Meals

Adding aroma, taste and color to your foods is a great way to jazz them up without using oil, salt or fat for flavor. They've been used for centuries to create culinary delights all over the world and they're now being added to food for health reasons.

Herbs are fresh or dried leaves of certain plants that are normally green in color. Spices, by definition, are the fruits, seeds, flowers, roots or barks of mostly tropically grown plants. They vary in color from black to brown or red.

Spices usually have a more intense flavor than herbs, but it's possible for one plant to provide both a spice and an herb. Plants which provide spices and herbs have been recorded as far back as the 1500s and some are medicinal in value.

People have been studying herbs and spices for centuries and now we have an abundance of selections from the most common to the most exotic – and most can be ordered online or found at your local health food or bulk food store.

As part of your mindful eating techniques, you'll want to add spices and herbs to bring out the color, taste and smell of your food. Your salt intake can be drastically cut with the use of herbs and spices and you can use many of them fresh or dried.

A few of the top spices and herbs you should be sure are in your kitchen for mindful cooking are basil, thyme, oregano, unrefined (coarse) salt, chili powder, cumin, garlic, cayenne, rosemary, black peppercorns (for grinding), sage, cinnamon, nutmeg and ginger.

With the above spices ready for use in your kitchen, you can make any meal sing with good flavor and good health. A word of caution: Avoid spice mixes. They usually contain salt and preservatives and could have been sitting on the shelf for quite some time so the ingredients have lost their intensity.

Slow Cookers and Blenders

The benefits of preparing meals with slow cookers and blenders include health and speed. You can use a slow cooker to prepare a meal in the morning and then enjoy it that evening without doing anything in-between.

A blender can whip up shakes and smoothies in seconds and you can use healthy fruits and veggies that will taste better than an ice cream shop when you're finished. Your kids will be begging for more and you don't have to tell them all the good things that are in it.

Slow cookers have been making a comeback lately and are being enjoyed for the ease and the mouth-watering aromas that make you hungry all day.

Now, you can purchase small slow cookers for one (or a couple) or large ones for family meals.

Soups and stews become more savory and meats can be cooked to fall-apart goodness and aroma with the use of herbs and spices for flavor. And, keep in mind that a slow cooker can turn some processed foods, such as canned tomatoes, into nutrition-packed products because of the slow cooking process (similar to the benefits you get from canning).

Other foods such as corn and spinach also release important nutrients while being heated. A recent study proved that the healthy carotenoid content (zeaxanthin and lutein) of frozen, fresh or canned corn are released during a slow cooking process.

Legumes such as lentils are also improved with heat – and they contain nutrients that aren't found in other food products. Also, when you heat meats at a low heat and in a bit of liquid, you can decrease the amount of cell-damaging (AGEs) compounds which can be produced by grilling or broiling.

Using a blender is another mindful method of preparing healthy and fast food. The benefits include ingesting more fiber from fruits and veggies, less raising of blood sugar than juicing, uses every bit of the ingredients (no waste), lets you prepare superfoods by using ingredients such as flax seeds, goji berries and chlorella during the blending process and is a filling way to eat a meal.

Blending is also an easy way to get your daily amount of vegetables and fruit, plus it's less time-consuming. Just pile on the kale, parsley, spinach, broccoli, some cilantro and other greens into the blender then drink your way to health.

Healthy fats are also easy to consume with a blender. Avocados, coconut milk, flax seed oil and extra virgin olive oil can be added to other ingredients in your blender to provide fats that are crucial to your brain, nerve, blood and cholesterol health.

When you're stressed for time, these two methods can save your sanity and provide exactly what you're looking for in a meal for yourself and those you love. They're just a couple more ways that you can take advantage of mindful eating in today's world.

Recipes for healthy blender and slow cooker meals abound, both online and in books. Take advantage of these two healthy and fast methods of preparing mindful meals for yourself and your family.

Meditation in the Kitchen

It may seem odd to see "meditation in the kitchen" as a mindful cooking technique, but when meditation becomes integrated into your daily life, it tends to be more meaningful – and what better place to bring peace into your life than the kitchen?

Meditation while preparing meals helps you explore your mind for the challenges you're facing and helps you pay special attention to the love and devotion you're putting into the preparation of each meal.

It can be a fun practice to think about each ingredient and each cooking process that goes into every recipe. Make it enjoyable rather than serious and intense. Tradition says that your emotions are transmitted from the chef to the food and to avoid contaminating your ingredients, you should think loving thoughts as you're cooking.

When you cook a meal in meditation and loving thoughts, you're not only providing food for your body – you're adding peace to your mind and spirit. Foods that are factory produced don't bring that element to the table.

That's why Mom's home cooking can't be replaced by Kentucky Fried Chicken or Taco Bell. Mom puts an element of meditation and love in her cooking that can't be duplicated. Enjoy the creativity and peace that can be found when cooking mindfully in your kitchen.

Chapter 4: Try New Recipes

Mindful eating isn't the type of eating regime where you must eat certain foods and only small quantities of those. In fact, it isn't a regime at all. It's a way to lose weight and get all the nutrition you need by simply changing recipes to make them healthier and cooking in new and innovative ways.

You'll never get bored with this type of eating because there's always something new to learn. And, it's incredibly easy to use mindful eating techniques to revamp old recipes and make them more nutritious and less caloric.

Most of us fixate on certain meals – especially when on diets – and never venture out to try other cuisine. There is an abundance of ethnic cuisines which are both healthy and would probably be new to your palate.

Using mindful eating techniques, you can let your experimentation into new foods run wild. You'll use a different combination of spices and herbs and try new ways of cooking such as using yogurt rather than sour cream or stir-frying rather than deep-fat frying.

One thing is for sure – you'll never get bored when using mindful eating techniques if you use them properly and with enthusiasm. This chapter contains ways you can spiff up your recipes and eating habits in healthier ways.

Mindful Eating – the Mediterranean Way

No diet or plan of eating has ever come along that is better for you and offers more of a variety of foods than Mediterranean-style dining. It's the ultimate mindful eating experience.

Countries around the Mediterranean Sea have long-produced a population which is healthier and more robust than the rest of the world. The lush and delicious bounty that the climate and soil produce provides a healthy abundance that keeps the surrounding people in a health class all their own.

Today, it's possible to have all the benefits of the Mediterranean way of life without actually living there. Transportation methods and the way we grow food provides much of the rest of the world with all the ingredients it needs to live a healthy lifestyle and enjoy food in a mindful manner.

The Mediterranean way of eating and living isn't simply a diet – it's a lifestyle. It combines healthy foods with activities and enjoying meals with family and friends rather than alone in front of the television or on the run.

Wine is also a part of the Mediterranean lifestyle, but it's imbibed in moderation. Scientists have long studied the Mediterranean lifestyle and have unequivocally dubbed it as the "healthiest in the world."

When you think of a table spread with an abundance of Mediterranean style food, think of such items as whole-grain pasta with veggies, Couscous, Greek salads filled with cheeses, greens, nuts and grains, Hummus, served with warm, whole-grain Pita and perhaps Spinach, sautéed with a hint of lemon juice.

Rather than eating on the run, a Mediterranean style meal can last for hours and each morsel of food is carefully and lovingly prepared and served. You may not be able to replicate all of the Mediterranean lifestyle in your own home, but you can bring in elements which can help you succeed with mindful eating and weight loss.

The Mediterranean diet plan is based on a pyramid which serves as a visual, universal guide (named the "gold standard") for eating a diet promoting good health for a lifetime. Health professionals and educators use this pyramid to help implement mindful eating habits with their patients.

The pyramid advocates consuming an abundance of food from plants, including grains, beans, fruits, nuts, vegetables and seed. Use olive oil as the principal source of fat, mostly replacing others such as margarine and fat.

Low-fat and non-fat cheeses and yogurt should be consumed moderately and fish and poultry eaten about twice per week. Lean, red can be eaten in moderation about once per month and red wine can be consumed daily with meals (2 glasses per day for men and 1 glass for women).

This pyramid has been tested, both epidemiologically and nutritionally for the past 50 years and has remained the main reason for the Mediterranean region enjoying the lowest rates of chronic diseases and a life expectancy far above most of the rest of the world.

It would be in your best interest, if you want to live a long and healthy life, to study the Mediterranean lifestyle and see how some of it can be adapted to your own life. Recipes and suggestions about how to shop are abundant both online and in books and magazines.

Other Healthy Ethnic Cuisines

Besides the Mediterranean-style cuisine and way of life, there are other ethnic cuisines you may want to try to get the most out of mindful eating techniques. Many of these recipes are full of health-restoring nutrients and are low in calories.

Traditional Japanese cuisine is one rich in fruits and vegetables which have been proven to fight cancer. Bok choy and mushrooms (shitake variety) are light and nutritious and can add interest to any meal.

On the island of Okinawa, the dietary practices are believed to be the reason why people tend to live over a 100 years of age. The Okinawan diet is rich in cancer-fighting foods such as vegetables and fruit and they're prepared in a stir-fry or using steam.

Miso Soup, tofu, tempeh, soybean cake (using fermented soybeans), edamame and seafood are typical at a Japanese/Okinawan meal. Most everything they consume are sources of zinc, folate, iron and potassium.

Indian cuisine is full of the aromatic spices that adds to the distinctive flavors of a diet rich in cancer-fighting and healing properties. Turmeric, curry's main ingredient is said to contain healing properties and powerful anti-inflammatory benefits.

Rates of the memory-robbing Alzheimer's disease are many times lower in India than in America. The rates are attributed to the fact that Indians consume at least 100 to 200 milligrams of curry on a daily basis. The benefits of turmeric are now being studied in many universities.

Other ingredients in a healthy Indian diet include lentils (folate and magnesium) and yogurt. Dal is a dish which is made from lentils, mixed with a combination of delicious Indian spices and often served as a side dish or snack.

Leisurely meals are often enjoyed in Italian tradition, with foods that aid digestion. The stars of this cuisine are tomatoes, garlic, basil, parsley, oregano and olive oil. High in lycopene, tomatoes are believed to prevent and protect women from breast cancer.

Cooked tomatoes such as tomato paste contain more than 20 milligrams in only a half-cup. Vitamins A and C are abundant in garlic and Italian herbs and olive oil is a power-food which assists in lowering cholesterol, preventing heart disease and burning unwanted fat cells.

Vietnamese dining means you'll be consuming vegetables and seafood cooked in water or broth rather than oil. Herbs are used extensively in cooking rather than heavy and unhealthy sauces. Mint, cilantro, red chili and Thai basil can help to aid digestion and have many anti-inflammatory qualities.

The fact that Vietnamese food is mostly cooked in water rather than frying in oils makes it lower in calories. Pho (pronounced "fuh") is one of the healthiest Vietnamese dishes and is made from broth and noodles, plus many highly antioxidant spices.

You may think of Mexican cuisine as high in calories and fat because of the offerings at most Mexican food restaurants. But, authentic Mexican food can slim you down and make you healthier.

Mexican soups, sauces based on tomato, beans and corn can protect women from breast cancer as well as Type 2 diabetes. If you're thinking of trying Mexican cuisine, stay away from the queso and chips.

You don't have to live on the West Coast of the United State to have the benefits of California cuisine. It's fresh and tasty and simply prepared – with plenty of low calorie, nutrient and mineral rich fruits and vegetables.

Local farmers' markets do a booming business and foods there taste better and are healthier for you than their processed counterparts. But, you likely have seasonal farmers' markets near your own home where you can purchase many wonderful items, including freshly baked, whole-grain bread.

Food from Spain can also whet your appetite for the healthy and unusual. Just avoid the sausages, laden with fat, fried foods which are popular tapas in Spain and stick with fresh seafood, olive oil and vegetables.

Dishes that are especially healthy from Spain include gazpacho (with lycopene and antioxidants) and paella (a rich mixture of rice, vegetables and seafood. Tapas are small offerings of food, where you get to sample a variety of deliciously prepared foods.

Thai cuisine is a growing trend in the West. Soups such as Tom Yung Gung may be helpful to fight cancer. It's a combination of shrimp, lemongrass, coriander and other tasty spices and herbs and has been scientifically found to contain properties which are 100 times more effective in fighting cancer tumor growth than other foods containing antioxidants.

Ginger, a main ingredient in Thai recipes, aids in digestion while lemongrass helps relieve cold and stomach symptom.

If you're experimenting with Thai recipes, avoid those with coconut milk which is high in calories and saturated fat.

Mindful Snacking Tips

Everyone has cravings and times when you've just got to have a snack to keep going – usually in the middle of the afternoon. Children crave after school snacks to keep their energy up until dinner time. But snacking is an area where too many calories may be consumed if you're not mindful about your choices.

The worst thing you could do is grab a snack from a vending machine which is usually filled with cookies, chips and candy bars. They're usually loaded with unhealthy fats and sodium, high in sugar content and low in important nutrients such as fiber. You can make much healthier choices.

Snacks can add as much as between 500 and 600 calories to your daily food intake and lead to weight gain and difficulty in controlling your blood glucose levels, which can lead to diabetes.

But, a healthy snack can provide you with extra nutrients and prevent hunger which may lead to binging and overeating. Some healthy snacks include nuts, vegetables, fruit and whole grains. Be sure to watch your portion size as many of these healthy snacks are relatively high in calories.

When you just can't resist grabbing a snack, try being mindful and rather than choosing a candy bar, grab a ¼ cup of roasted nuts or half a frozen banana or 15 grapes rather than an ice cream bar.

Other suggestions include plain Greek yogurt with berries mixed in or baked tortilla chips with a small serving of guacamole rather than the fried tortilla chips with highly processed nacho cheese.

Mindful snack choices also include a piece of light string cheese with a piece of fruit, peanut butter dipped with celery and carrots or freshly cut veggies with Hummus or light Ranch dressing for dipping.

South American food is diverse, but most all countries in South America use fresh vegetables and fruits combined with quinoa – a high protein grain. They typically consume a meal of rice and beans which combine to make a perfect protein.

Many of the above cuisines have been "Westernized" and don't contain the health benefits that they were originally designed to have. You can adapt healthy recipes in your repertoire to become classic ethnic dishes and give yourself and your family a change from the usual dinner fare.

Super Foods You Can Add to Any Recipe

You may already be aware of the recent trend of adding super healthy foods such as kale, quinoa and Greek yogurt. Others you may not know about include Chia seeds which contain as much protein as many nuts and also provide alpha-linolenic acid, the plant-based fat (omega-3) and other benefits like fiber and protein.

Toss the Chia seeds into pancake mix, oatmeal and sprinkle over cereal to give your meal a crunch and a big dose of healthy to your body. Chia seeds are becoming a mega-food fad, but have been around since the days of the Aztecs.

Explore the benefits of other super-healthy ingredients such as coconut flour (full of fiber and gluten-free) and Skyr (Icelandic yogurt) you can add to your mindful eating recipes and reap all the benefits they offer – plus help with the weight loss you desire.

.

Chapter 5: Adopt Mindful Eating HAbits

What is a mindful eating habit? Does it mean you don't allow yourself to eat certain things or to eat less of it? The best way to define mindful eating is to define what mindless eating is.

You've likely experienced mindless eating when watching a football game while eating pizza in front of the television. All of a sudden the pizza (and a couple of drinks) is gone and you don't remember eating it.

Or – you ate your lunch at work in front of the computer and at the end of the day, you don't remember what you ate or when. Those are mindless eating examples. Now, you'll learn about mindful eating and how it can help you become healthier and lose unwanted pounds.

Intentions of Mindful Eating

Developing healthy eating habits and weight loss are the true intentions of mindful eating. A constant awareness of your present state of hunger and how food is affecting your body (is it healthy or unhealthy?) are part of the reasons why mindful eating can make you successful in all things involving food.

Knowing about your own hunger cues to see if you're still hungry – or simply want more to eat because it tastes good or you're used to being fuller – is one method of using mindful eating as a weight loss tool.

Mindful eating also addresses the attention of enjoying the food you consume. You'll learn what your non-hunger cues are for eating and also about your hunger cues which alert you to eat nourishing foods which will alleviate your hunger and be good and healthy for your body.

Using mindful eating techniques, you'll learn how to deal with the discomfort you might experience from smaller portions and how to know if you're eating from habit or actual hunger.

There is a scale you can use to measure your hunger cues. If your hunger level is at a 10, you're miserably stuffed – whereas a 0 means that you're at starvation. Mindful eating advocates that you should only eat when your hunger level hits a 4 and stop when you reach a 6. It's something to keep in mind when planning your meals for the most effectiveness.

Another intention of mindful eating is to choose other avenues other than eating to meet your emotional and physical needs. Many of us eat based on emotional turmoil and that leads to overeating and weight gain.

Learning to choose your meals based on both enjoyment and nourishment value is a big part of mindful eating. When you learn to do this, you're going to be more satisfied with your choices and get the most in nutritional value from the foods you choose.

Another intention of mindful eating is providing you with the energy you need to live the life you visualize. Imagine having the energy you need to achieve the goals and create the physique you desire.

Mindful eating can provide answers to all of these intentions – and more. Finally, you'll be able to develop a healthy relationship with food and eating.

No longer will you eat to satisfy emotional needs, but you'll be more mindful about eating to provide your body with nutrition and energy it needs to function properly.

Questions and Answers to Help Your Mindful Eating Journey

Can you go back for seconds if you're still hungry? How can mindful eating help you break old habits of eating for pleasure and based on emotions? Mindful eating is a method of consuming food where you're always in the present moment.

At first, you may analyze your every thought and feeling. Am I really hungry? What do I really want to eat? Mindful eating techniques will teach you how to recognize hunger cues and get rid of old habits which don't work for you anymore – replacing them with good habits that do work.

Many of us are unhealthy and overweight because we stuff our faces with fast food and food that contains no nutrients. We become addicted to the rush that fatty and fried foods give us, so we eat those foods mindlessly as a way to cope with constant hunger rather than choosing healthy foods that would really help.

Other questions that people have when thinking about trying mindful eating techniques include:

How do I get over cravings for fatty foods?

It may take a while to get over your cravings, but by replacing those unhealthy foods with foods that are much more filling and nutritious for your body, you'll find that your system will adjust and you'll feel better with your new choices.

How do I find time for preparing healthy meals?

With mindful eating techniques, you'll learn that healthy meals can be prepared and enjoyed without compromising on your valuable time and efforts. Slow cookers, blenders and steamers are just a few of the mindful eating cooking methods which can be used to save time.

At what point do I know to stop eating?

There is a scale used for pain measurement which can also be used for measuring your hunger. The scale is based on 1 through 10 –10 being the point where you're really stuffed and 1 being the point that you think you're starving. Take a minute to analyze your hunger point before eating more.

How do I overcome wanting to enjoy my meals while watching my favorite television shows?

Make it a point to spiff up your dining table and make it inviting for you and your family. Soft music in the background and flowers on the table can go a long way in making it an inviting and peaceful place to enjoy your meals.

How do I avoid social overeating?

If you're at a restaurant or someone's house, choose items from the menu or table that are low in calories. If that's not an option, eat a small portion – or ask for a doggie bag to take some home.

If you get stuck on a mindful eating question, just use your common sense and hunger cues to lead you on the path you need to take. Don't fret if you indulge in "mindless" eating once in a while. It's difficult to stop eating while watching television or at your desk and you may not have a choice on busy days.

Begin with a day a week where you practice the art of mindful eating and use the other days to practice and learn. Keep nutrition and true hunger at the center of your mindful eating journey and you'll eventually notice the difference.

Replacing Mindless Eating Habits with Mindful Eating Habits

It's helpful to use what is known as the "stepladder" approach to mindful eating until it's a true part of your daily routine. You may want to begin with replacing a simple habit such as snacking on unhealthy foods with the habit of snacking on foods such as those recommended in Chapter 4, "Mindful Snacking Tips."

You won't become a mindful eater overnight and replace all your bad eating habits with good ones, but you can begin to be present in mind, body and spirit when you do make choices about the foods you're going to consume.

Taking the process slow will have greater chances of it sticking and your accomplishments will multiply until the mindful eating habits become a part of your daily routine just like brushing your teeth.

There are some easy and effortless ways you can begin to replace bad, old eating habits with good and nutritious ones. One way is to carefully plan your meals for the week.

Shopping for and stocking up on all the ingredients you'll need for your snacks and meals will give you a head start on developing newer and healthier habits and getting rid of the old ones.

Be aware of every morsel of food you put in your mouth and also how it's prepared. After you place the food on a plate, take small bites and savor each mouthful, chewing carefully before swallowing.

If you ordinarily eat too fast, practice a slower method by putting your knife and fork down between bites. Other methods include using chopsticks and only putting on your plate what you plan to consume.

Keep your mental attitude positive. Your mental attitude has everything to do with your enthusiasm and consumption of food. If you're nervous or upset, you may consume more than planned. Before a meal, make an attempt to become calm and serene so your meal and the digestion process will proceed smoothly.

If you've dieted to lose weight most of your life, try dieting to get healthy. Make you goal that of being and obtaining the best body possible. That will help you overcome your obsession with weight loss and get you to be more mindful of what you're eating that will help improve and maintain your health.

Make Dieting a Thing of the Past

By making mindful eating part of your daily routine, you won't think of yourself as "on a diet" anymore. Rather, you'll be striving to get the most out of your food without causing problems in other areas of your life.

Mindful eating isn't dieting. It's a way of life that uses your mind and intuitive skills to develop a healthy relationship with food and your mind and body.

Diets of the past only use external methods such as counting calories and weight scales, whereas mindful eating focuses on your own self and internal cues of hunger.

Problems such as binging are often solved with mindful eating techniques because you learn to recognize hunger cues and you'll also be eating enough good food to satisfy your mind and body.

Healthy living promotes a spiritual and intellectual outlook on food that isn't at all like the old dieting methods of starving yourself by taking a militaristic stance on what and how you dine.

Using mindful eating techniques will teach you how to eat when you're hungry and stop eating when you're satisfied. You'll also learn to love the taste of healthy foods and avoid the taste of unhealthy foods because of how they make you feel.

Social overeating becomes a thing of the past because you'll learn how to eat with your mind rather than urges when you're socializing. As a result, you'll begin to enjoy your eating experiences more and crave less.

You'll also begin to enjoy life more because you will become more present in other areas of your life such as relationships and work. Your eating times will be events to look forward to rather than dread and you'll notice how your food intake affects your energy levels during the day.

Through the act of mindful eating, you'll feel more like exercising and preparing healthy meals that both you and your family and friends will enjoy. You may not ever become a gourmet chef, but you can learn to appreciate the various ingredients that go into making a tasty meal.

Dos and Don'ts of Mindful Eating

There are a few hard and fast rules that you should always think about when adopting mindful eating techniques. One is to begin small – perhaps with a snack during the day. Make it a snack that you choose for its health benefits and taste.

Don't multitask when you're eating. It may not always be possible, but attempt to set aside one meal during the week where you set the table and prepare a nutritious meal. Block out all distractions and simply enjoy the food and peace of the meal.

Eat at a table rather than in your bed or in front of the television set or computer. Only then will you be able to give your food the attention it needs to make an impact on your eating habits.

Pay attention to your meal. Notice the color, texture and all aspects of how it looks and tastes. Make your meals beautiful by using herbs, spices and garnishes that will set it apart from the usual fare.

Take small bites and chew your food well. You'll be surprised how important this is to aid digestion and help you focus on the delicious sensations that the food provides. Also, pay attention to the aroma and bitterness or sweetness that you taste and smell.

Sharing a meal with loved ones is an important part of mindful eating. In today's world, it can be challenging to get everyone together for a meal at home, but try incorporating at least one day per week for eating a meal together and talk and share your memories of the day – and the delicious meal you've prepared.

You don't have to prepare huge meals, but do purchase the best ingredients you can. Fresh fruits and vegetables go much farther in taste than processed ones. You'll enjoy it more and be much more satisfied at the end of the meal.

When you embark on a journey of mindful eating, you'll be creating a lifestyle for yourself that's simple and fun and makes any eating experience worthwhile and enjoyable.

Chapter 6: Familiarize Yourself with Fast Food Options

It's simply a given – sometimes, you're going to be faced with the prospect of ordering fast food no matter how much thought and effort you've given to adopting mindful eating techniques.

You need to know your options so you won't be forced to order a salad or a dreaded double cheeseburger with fries. You want to order wisely, so as not to mess up your low calorie intake that you've adhered to so well all week.

When eating at fast food places, beware of the "healthy" options advertised that can pack a whopping amount of calories. But, there are options that will provide some macronutrients without also loading you up on calories or sugar and salt.

Moderation is key when dining at fast food establishments and there are some other things you should keep in mind. Keep lunches under 500 calories and choose a meal that carries at least 10 grams of protein.

Keep it low in sodium (less than 1,000 milligrams). That's about the best you can hope for at a fast food place, so be sure and look for other options if you have high blood pressure.

Low sugar content is also a must (less than 20 grams) and trans fats should be avoided at all cost. Trans fats can cause heart disease, so look for options which offer 0 grams of trans fat.

Choose bottled water rather than a sugary drink and don't succumb to fries or other sides that can add calories and other harmful ingredients. Mindful eating advocates that you should eat what you want, so if you really feel like a cheeseburger, get it. Just try to make healthier decisions during other meals of the day.

Best Drive Through Options

No matter what drive through establishment you choose, try to keep your options as small as possible and avoid sides that can shatter your good intentions. Now, some fast food restaurants (including McDonald's) offer salads that are under 500 calories, but beware of the dressings which are high in sodium and sugar.

McDonald's also offers an Artisan Grilled Chicken Sandwich, full of protein and some veggies and it comes in at about 360 calories. It's a good option if you find yourself with kids or friends who insist on McDonald's.

You can find a Fresco Steak Burrito Supreme (with black beans) for 430 calories or a Fresco Chicken Soft Taco with pinto beans and cheese for under 330 calories. But, both of these options contain some saturated fat.

Even Dunkin' Donuts can provide you with a tuna salad sandwich on an English muffin for only 390 calories or an Egg White Veggie Wake-Up Wrap with hash browns for breakfast weighing in at only 350 calories. Again, some saturated fat is involved.

Subway touts healthy options in its advertisements and you can get a 6-inch Club sandwich on 9-grain wheat bread with veggies and sweet onion sauce (it also comes with apple slices).

Or choose the Oven roasted chicken salad with veggies and honey mustard dressing (with a yogurt parfait). These are each 400 calories.

If you're a fan of Starbuck's, choose from the chicken and black bean salad bowl (450 calories) or the chicken and hummus bistro box that comes with hummus, grilled chicken, grape tomatoes, cucumber and pita bread (and a banana) for only 450 calories.

Burger King won't be outdone with its Whopper Jr that comes with no mayo, but a few onion rings –all for under 450 calories. Or, you can opt for the veggie burger with apple slices for just 440 calories.

Panera has become a popular option for the lunch crowd and you can choose from the Power Mediterranean Chicken Salas with baked potato chips that will only cost you 430 calories – or, a half turkey breast sandwich on whole grain bread that comes with a low-fat vegetable soup for under 400 calories.

Healthy options are also available at KFC, where you can order four hot wings with corn for only 380 calories or a grilled breast of chicken with mashed potatoes for just 310 calories.

It's still best to avoid fast food if possible. There is some saturated fat in all of the above options. But, if you're on the run and can't avoid it, some options exist that won't put you in a tailspin from mindful eating.

How to Avoid Fast Food Traps

Although it's very tempting to succumb to fast food when you're running short of time, the kids are hungry and there's nothing in the fridge at home. But one look at the average calorie count and harmful ingredients (especially saturated fats) contained in most fast food meals and you may think twice about alternatives.

One alternative to stopping by for fast food is to make a quick trip into your local supermarket. You're in luck if you have a Trader Joe's or Central Market nearby because you can purchase fresh salads, fruits and deli items (including sandwiches) that are pre-made and most even come with plastic eating utensils. Grab a bottle of water and you're good to go.

Consider packing a cooler or lunch container with leftovers. Most people have leftovers lurking in their fridge. Grab a container and some ice and throw in some grapes, cheese and other munchies to tide you over until you can get a good meal.

This is an especially good idea if you or a family member has food allergies. You never know if there will be a place in the town you're traveling to that can accommodate your needs.

If possible, take your lunch or breakfast to a picnic table in a park or roadside rest area and get some fresh air and let the kids run around to release some of that pent up energy from riding the car when traveling.

Always keep snacks such as fruit, cheese and veggies in the refrigerator so you can grab them on the go.

If you have time in the morning, a well-planned smoothie can be much more satisfying and healthier than a trip to McDonald's for an Egg McMuffin and hashbrowns.

Another reason to avoid fast food restaurants is the amount of sodium that's contained in most of their offerings. Sodium is the single-most harmful food for heart disease, hypertension and other ailments that can put you in an early grave.

Most at risk for developing health problems because of high consumption of salt are people over 50 years of age, those who already have hypertension issues, those who suffer from diabetes and the African American population.

When you consume too much sodium, your body retains water you drink so it can dilute the sodium. This causes an increase of fluid surrounding your blood cells and also increases the amount of blood in your bloodstream so that your heart and blood vessels have to work overtime.

Over a period of time, your heart can fail because of the added work and your kidneys, aorta and bones may also be damaged – all due to excess salt in your diet. A part of the mindful eating process should definitely be to lower the consumption of sodium in your diet.

This means that you should do everything possible to avoid fast food restaurants which are some of the main culprits for too much salt. You're also missing most of the main vitamins and minerals found in fresh foods that you prepare yourself as opposed to the dietary disasters that you have to order at the fast food establishments.

Another fast-food trap to avoid is salads that sound healthy, but which load you with calories, saturated fats and sodium galore.

You can add some dressing to a healthy salad, but most of the dressings found at fast food places are high in calories and sodium content.

How Fast Food Affects Your Body

Mindful eating tells you that food is to be considered fuel for your body – but that you should enjoy preparing and eating your food to get the full, healthy effect. Fast food isn't all bad, but most contains huge amounts of sugar, unhealthy fats, carbs and sodium.

They mostly offer no nutritional value whatsoever and bring risks of chronic health problems such as diabetes, stroke and heart disease. Now, children are the unlucky recipients of taking in more calories in fast food places than at home.

A constant diet of fast food can affect many areas of the body. The cardiovascular and digestive systems are two ways most fast food can harm your body. When your digestive system breaks down the many carbs you eat in a fast food meal, they turn into sugar, which is then released into your blood stream.

Your pancreas and other areas of the body have to work overtime to keep the insulin levels within normal range and can lead to failure of organs and chronic diseases that can lead to death.

The respiratory system (lungs) can also suffer when you become obese from too much of the foods that have no nutritional value. Asthma or rhinitis (a constant runny nose or congestion) is prevalent in children who have a consistent diet of fast foods.

The skin and skeletal structures of the body can be harmed by trans fats and processed chocolate. Carbs may cause acne in teenagers or increase blood levels. Eczema (inflamed skin) is also a side effect of eating too much fast food.

The bones are affected by sodium. Too much may cause osteoporosis, a thinning of the bones, making them fragile and prone to break. Your teeth are also subjected to harm from fast food. Acids from high carb/sugary foods can destroy the enamel of your teeth and cause other health problems.

Your central nervous system can be highly affected by fast food such as commercial breads and other baked goods such as pizza and doughnuts. New studies also link fast food with depression, indicating that over 51 percent of those who eat a consistent diet of fast foods were more likely to become depressed than those who didn't.

Fast (junk) foods are also linked to memory and learning losses. Studies showed that rats given a diet of half fat calories had trouble making their way through a maze that they had previously learned.

Obesity and all the problems which can come from it can also be linked to diets of fast food. We've become a fast-food consuming society rather than using mindful eating techniques that could save our health and prolong our lives.

Some Quick Drive-Through Tips

There are some definite strategies involved when contemplating eating from a fast food restaurant. These strategies will help you avoid the traps that can put you over the top on calories and harmful ingredients. If you must eat a meal on the run, they're good strategies to know.

The first strategy is to pay attention to so-called, "health halos." These are dishes which are advertised as healthy for you, but that can be laden with unnecessary calories. Be sure to read the list of nutritional values before ordering. You might be better off with a hamburger than a salad.

You hold knowledge in the palm of your hand if you have a cell phone. Now, you can download a Fast Food Calorie Counter which offers restaurants and over 9,000 items in various places.

Order from the kids' menu. Junior burgers are smaller and contain less calories than the Whopper. Look for places that use egg whites or lettuce wraps. Even Dunkin' Donuts offers all-day breakfast choices that are nutritious.

Watch the condiments and salad dressing options. Many are laden with calories that would be easy to avoid. For example, a packet of ketchup only contains 10 calories, whereas packets of honey mustard or barbeque sauce may contain as many as 60 calories.

If you must have fries with your burger, choose the small or medium variety rather than super-sized. In fact, avoid "super-sized" anything on a fast food menu. Also, look for broiled, grilled or roasted when it comes to meat, but avoid the cheese and rich sauces.

Water, unsweetened tea or low-fat milk should be your drink of choice. Keep in mind that a large carbonated drink packs at least 400 calories and is bad for you to boot. And, a milkshake can set you back over 1,000 calories.

If you love burgers, get your fix by choosing the smallest size available and specify no cheese, but double the veggies. Never add "special sauce," or salt and also avoid may which can add up to 200 calories on your sandwich.

Chili and soups can also be good choices at those fast food places that offer them. Sides can also be negotiated by choosing a small salad or a fruit salad rather than fries with your burger.

Use the mindful eating techniques you've learned in this book to make better choices, both at home and when dining out. Soon, you'll begin to notice subtle changes such as better mood, loss of unwanted pounds and a satisfaction of knowing that you're eating healthier – and actually liking it.

Product Reviews

In this chapter are product one-page reviews, along with a link to each product referenced in the book. If you purchase from those links, I'll get a small commission which will be much appreciated.

500 Heart Healthy Slow Cooker Recipes

If there's one thing we all understand when it comes to eating, it's comfort food. These kinds of food invoke warm memories and they make us feel better when we're happy and when we're down. It's why they're called comfort foods - they console us.

These kinds of foods can easily sabotage a weight loss plan. Plus, they can be bad for your heart. But if you know how you can tweak the foods you love to make them heart healthy and help you lose weight, then you can still have the comfort foods that you love.

That's one of the reasons why a cookbook like **500 Heart-Healthy Slow Cooker Recipes: Comfort Food Favorites That Both Your Family and Doctor Will Love** (http://amzn.to/1J5YvKI) will be one that you'll refer to time and again.

Not only will you be able to have the comfort foods that you enjoy but you'll be able to have them in a convenient and healthy way. By using a crockpot, you can your meals waiting for you when you're hungry. This can help to cut down on the urge to grab foods that aren't as good for you.

Normally, if you prepare foods in the slow cooker, you'd end up with foods that you'd be better off not eating. It can be easy to think you can use any recipe in the slow cooker and have it be good for you. But many of those foods can contain amounts of fat and sodium that are too high.

But by using this 480-page book, you can find dishes that are healthy and won't contribute to high blood pressure or raise cholesterol levels. The recipes in the cookbook are fast to make but taste like they were complicated creations.

You'll find main dishes like chili or Thai chicken that you can serve up but you'll also be able to find recipes that include vegetables you can make in the slow cooker. There are recipes for beef as well as for pork and lamb.

If you're not a fan of eating meat, you'll also find some delicious tasting meatless recipes. There are recipes for appetizers so you can have healthy food for family get-togethers or parties.

Plus, the book contains recipes that will enable you to use the slow cooker to make breakfast dishes or desserts. The book is great for anyone who wants to lose weight but it's also good for people who need to be on a low sodium, low fat diet for health reasons.

Using this cookbook is a heart friendly way of having the comfort foods that you want and you'll still end up losing weight to boot!

Crockpot Programmable Cooker

If you're one of those people who eat out of exhaustion – who come home bone tired, and reach for unhealthy snack foods, rather than home cooked, healthy meals – then you might want to consider investing in an affordable crockpot that does most of the work for you.

Having a crockpot is almost like having a personal chef in some ways. The cooking is done with a hands-off approach. You simple put in the ingredients, set it to the right temperature, and remove the food once it's done!

Slow cookers help you avoid fattening, fried foods as well. And you can cook for one – or for a whole family, providing delicious, home-cooked meals and steering clear of the fast food routine.

The **Crock-Pot Programmable Cook and Carry Oval Slow Cooker** (http://amzn.to/1n458mP) is a large crockpot that allows you to cook for up to seven people. It's programmable, so you can cook for half an hour or up to twenty hours, depending on your choice of meals.

Once your meal is done, the cooker automatically turns itself to a warm setting, simply keeping your food at the right temperature for whenever your meal is ready to be consumed.

The lid on the crockpot locks, keeping all messes at bay, and when the meal is complete, you can lift the oval-shaped stoneware out of the cooker and place it right on your table for easy serving.

There are dozens of healthy crockpot cookbooks you can get to learn how to shave off calories and prepare more nutritious meals for your family. And just because you're busy, you'll no longer have an excuse to ditch your diet – because a crockpot makes it so easy to stick to your plan.

When the meal is finished, you can unplug the cooker and after it's cooled, wash it down with a soft cloth and soapy water. You can put the lid and stoneware in the dishwasher.

The crockpot is also portable, so if you're attending a family function or office party and want to bring along a healthy alternative, you can do it easily with a locking lid that won't spill the contents of your meal as you travel.

Crockpot cooking is a wonderful alternative to fried and heavy sauced meals. You get the rich flavor of a home cooked meal, with a fraction of the calories. You can cook once and have leftovers, or cook a new meal every day if you want to!

Eat Out, Eat Well

When you're at home, healthy eating is something that's fairly easy to do, even if you're eating comfort foods. There are ways you can make comfort foods low fat and good for you. But when you eat out, there are all sorts of things in the foods that can sabotage your healthy eating plan.

Many restaurant foods are high in calorie, packed with sodium, and loaded with saturated fats. So what ends up happening with a lot of people is they either skip restaurant eating altogether when they want to eat healthy or they count it as an "off the wagon" day and eat whatever. You don't have to sacrifice healthy eating when you eat out as long as you know what to look for.

In the book *Eat Out, Eat Well: The Guide to Eating Healthy in Any Restaurant* (http://amzn.to/1n45gms) by Hope Warshaw, you can learn how to make dining out part of a healthy eating plan. Regardless of whether you eat out weekly or not, you can learn how to locate the healthy choices that most restaurants do offer.

Just because a restaurant claims something is healthy, doesn't mean it is. For example, you would think that having a salad is a low calorie, low fat meal. But that depends on what the restaurant puts on the salad. Some restaurant sauces and dressings can add hundreds of calories, a ton of fat grams and an entire day's portion of sodium.

This book is perfect for people who want to eat healthy but it's also a great guide for people who are struggling with diabetes. It can show you what food choices to make that will help keep your glucose numbers from spiking into an unhealthy range from a meal.

Plus, the book can help show which foods you can choose at restaurants that are good for someone who wants to pay attention to heart health. As an added bonus, if you're trying to watch what you eat so that you can lose weight and still eat out, the book can help you with that as well.

You'll be able to choose healthy foods from fast food menus as well as foods from more upscale restaurants. The book offers some suggested meal choices as well as what size you should order in that particular meal.

The book shows consumers what they need to watch out for in foods when dining out and it also shows how you can ask for certain things to make your meal healthier. If you have a child who has diabetes, the book can help guide you toward what foods to order that's healthy for him. It also has a portion dealing with eating out when you have celiac disease or problems with gluten.

Fiesta 9-Inch Luncheon Plate

In the 1960s and 70s, serving sizes were a mere fraction of what they are today. The servings we are fed (or feed ourselves) on today's enormous plates are enough to feed an entire family – far too much for one person.

If you're concerned about your health, or want to shed some fat from your frame, you can easily make one simple tweak and begin losing weight without even trying. It's all has to do with which dinnerware you buy.

The **Fiesta 9-Inch Luncheon Plate** (http://amzn.to/1n45n1n) is one that mimics the servings from days gone by – the days when our waists were thinner, when diabetes hadn't yet spiraled out of control for the majority of the population – when fewer people battled with weight demons.

This is an individual plate that you can purchase for under $9 that will help whittle your waist, simply by forcing you to stop and make a decision of whether or not you're going to reload the plate with food after you've finished the initial serving.

It limits the size of your initial servings to a proper amount. These plates are sold as singles, so if you live alone, you're not forced to buy an entire 16-piece set that will just go to waste.

Although the plates are ceramic, they've been vitrified. They feel like a smooth, glass surface and yet they're not going to break easily on you or chip and look outdated quickly. In fact, they're backed with a warranty that replaces the plate if they chip within five years.

You want to start using the plate right away – for breakfast, lunch and dinner. You can buy them in a variety of beautiful colors, including sage, slate, cobalt, black, white, ivory, tangerine, sunflower, turquoise, lemongrass, paprika, plum, scarlet, and lapis.

When you've finished your smaller meal, simply put it in the dishwasher and clean it for next time. These plates are so durable, they can be used both in a microwave *and* in an oven if you want to reheat last night's leftovers. You can even put this plate in the freezer for storing certain dishes if you want!

At first, you may find it uncomfortable eating from a plate that you would typically consider the size of a bread or salad plate. Now, you're using that same size as your full dinner plate!

But this is the process that really makes you listen to your hunger cues and ask yourself the question, "Am I really still hungry, or am I just wanting to eat?" The Fiesta 9-Inch Luncheon Plates will provide an element of mindfulness to your meals that keeps things uncomplicated.

George Foreman Grill

When it comes to shedding fat and building lean muscle, grilling your foods is one of the best ways to consume protein and flavor up nutritious vegetables, too! But grilling outdoors can be such a pain.

The *George Foreman Grill* (http://amzn.to/1J5YczA) is an indoor alternative that allows you to cook any meal, any time of the day without all the hassle. You simply plug the grill in, place your meat or vegetables or other foods on the grill, and close the lid until it's done.

With a grill like this, you can cook up to four servings, so you're not missing out on much of the space that a larger outdoor grill gives you. Plus, the foods cook fast. The current model has improved cooking speeds of 35% over the prior versions.

Meats cook in a mere ten-minute timeframe – perfect for those hurrying out the door or coming home from work hungry, but not wanting to fill the void with empty calorie foods. And it can serve the entire family at once, too.

The grill comes will grill plates built into it that you can remove and wash separately, making it very convenient for clean-up and re-use. This grill comes in a black color, but you can get white or red, too.

You can also get a larger grill that serves up to five people at once. Or, if you'd prefer to downsize and take up less space on your counter, you can get a two person serving as well.

The grill plates have a durable, nonstick surface. But even for the cleaning you do have to do, there are George Foreman grill sponges you can get that make cleanup even easier.

What makes the George Foreman Grill such a healthy alternative? Aside from the fact that you're not breading and frying your meat cuts, the fat from your meat selection drains out – leaving you with the leanest option possible.

For those of you who have a big family and want to cook a variety of foods for a larger group of people, there's another George Foreman Grill that serves up to eight people. This option also has variable temperature control, not just the "plug in and cook" option.

You can stay on a low carb or low calorie diet with ease using a George Foreman Grill, and the best way to do that is to choose lean, boneless cuts of thin meat and season it for taste.

Gourmia Electric Digital Air Fryer

Fried foods always taste so good. But they're not very healthy for you, nor do they help you lose weight or keep toned when pounds are a factor in your life. Many people turn to alternative cooking methods, such as baking or steaming foods, but there's another form of cooking that's taking the diet industry by storm for its amazing health benefits – and it's called air frying!

When you cook in a gadget like the **Gourmia Electric Digital Air Fryer** (http://amzn.to/1n45VEw) you're able to have succulent fried chicken, crisp, warm French fries, and restaurant-quality onion rings without having to tell everyone you *fell off the wagon*.

Air frying keeps food crisp on the outside and moist on the inside, and it does it all without you having to add fattening oil to the mix. With this particular air fryer, you're given a slew of add-on components that help you make healthier meals.

You can use these accessories to turn the air fryer into a baker, griller, steamer, roaster and more. When you're done, clean-up is a cinch because it's all made of non-stick elements that you can remove quickly and easily.

How does an air fryer work? It circulates heated air around your food so that it's cooked without having to rely on oil to do the job. It also cooks faster. Your meal could be done in 60% less time than it would take to cook using a different method.

The eleven accessories that come with the air fryer include tongs to help you handle the foods, a crisp and fry basket, pans you can bake and steam in, a rotating rotisserie as well as a basket for it, steamer racks for both high and low broiling, a mesh filter made of steel, and a rack for kabobs.

Consumers love making healthy meals using the air fryer to create stir fried foods, health-conscious kabobs and more. You can also do other things, such as defrost your food using the air fryer, or turn on a specialty mode for items like pizzas.

What's the difference between an air fryer and a microwave oven? In terms of food quality during cooking – a lot! A microwave cooks your food from the inside out. So by the time it's on your plate, the inside is dry and the outside hasn't had time to get crisp while locking in moisture.

With an air fryer, it's heating the food from the outside in, forming a nice, crisp layer to seal in juices and keep food just the way you like it. Air frying is definitely an improvement in healthy cooking – the question for you is, will you be able to decide which dish you want to cook first in it?

Intuitive Eating

There's no doubt about it that chronic dieting isn't fun. Besides not being fun, it's not really good for your body to be in a state of continual dieting. There's a way that you can break free from chronic dieting, eat great foods, and still lose weight.

That method is through intuitive eating. This is the practice which basically means you pay attention to your body's hunger signals rather than trying to make food fit into your life. You allow your body's signals to guide you.

The *Intuitive Eating* (http://amzn.to/1J5YVR3) book is a guide which can help dieters learn how to shed the negative view of themselves that dieting has given them. Through the use of the book, you can learn how to quell the negative emotions and give food its proper place in your life.

You'll learn how to stop the blame game and quit beating yourself up when you can't seem to say no to food. You'll learn how to let go of dieting. In the process, you'll discover that food has never been the problem, that dieting is the culprit behind not only weight gain - but also behind making dieters feel badly about their efforts.

Through the help of the book, you'll learn about healthy eating by saying goodbye to going on a diet. You'll learn how to have food without a diet using food to control your emotions.

You'll also go on an inner reflection to discover how and why you eat. This is your eating personality and it can help you to uncover what your struggles are with food.

Instead of feeling bad about eating and dreading yet another diet filled with should and should nots, you'll be able to enjoy food once again. You'll be able to break the emotional eating habit even if it's something that's held you captive for years.

By using the ten principles outlined in the book, you'll be able to feel your hunger and hear what your body is saying to you. Some of these principles include things like letting go of dieting, loving your body and learning how you can respect it when your body lets you know it's full.

Saying goodbye to how you previous saw food will allow you to open up a new way of viewing food that's healthy and can lead to a natural weight loss. Since food habits and the way we view eating can be passed down to children in the family, the book also has a section where it covers how to raise kids who know the principles of intuitive eating. This 368-page book was written by nutritionists and can help anyone change their eating habits for the better.

Precise Portion Plates

One of the toughest things about learning how to lose weight through proper nutrition is portion control. Even when you're eating lower calorie foods, if your portions are too big, weight loss will be difficult.

The **Precise Portion Plates** (http://amzn.to/1J5Z1Zb) that you can get online help fix this common problem. Not everyone has (or wants to rely on) a food scale to measure out every single meal they consume.

The plates make this a simpler task, and they're still accurate in terms of helping you watch how much you eat. The plates are made of BPA-free plastic, so they deliver added health protection from harmful chemicals.

Each plate has three areas. One is for your vegetables (not the starchy kind, of course). One is where you put your lean cuts of meat. And the third is for your grain foods, or a bit of starch if you want to include that in your meal plan.

You can get the plates in sets of two or four, and there are two other ways you can use Precise Portion products, too! One is by getting the Lunch Bag and Travel Pack combo. If you eat on the go, you'll appreciate the way you can add a convenient lid to these plates and carry them with you wherever you go – to the office, on a picnic – anywhere!

The lids won't leak, and you can bring them home, put them in the dishwasher, and even microwave with them. They're not just for adults, either. Your kids can use them for school lunches or field trips, too.

If you just want the lunch bag, you can get that separately, and it will hold your portion control plate along with an ice pack. It even has a shoulder strap to help you carry it around.

Eating with the healthy portion control plates helps you get your metabolism revved up – so you burn fat faster and keep shedding pounds or maintaining a healthy weight once you reach it.

The Precise Portion Plates are sold in different variations, too. You can purchase a lifestyle system set that includes porcelain china with a design that's beautiful, yet informative to help you stay on track.

Hey also sell a "show and tell" type of plate for kids to use. It's a BPA-free plastic design that little ones have fun learning with. And if you're conscious about the ecosystem, you might want the compostable bamboo disposable portion plates that they sell.

Ronco Rotisserie

One nutritional element that experts will tell you to focus on while trying to lose weight is protein. Protein not only helps you feel full, longer – but it also helps your body build the muscles it needs to rev up your metabolism and keep you lean.

But eating meat can often mean ingesting unhealthy options, such as battered and fried foods. The **Ronco Rotisserie oven** (http://amzn.to/1J5Z5bo) is a wonderful alternative that helps you add plenty of lean protein to your dishes, without the added calories.

You can use the oven for a variety of fowl meals, such as turkeys, hens, ducks or chickens. But you can also use it for other cuts of meat as well, depending on your personal tastes.

You don't have to do main meat dishes, either. The oven is perfect for whipping up some healthy appetizers or desserts, too. You can cook so many dishes in it – from burgers and steaks to fish or even vegetables.

If you do go with rotisserie chicken, then you'll be using this self-basting machine to provide you with tons of nutrients, including niacin, phosphorous, potassium, zinc, B vitamins, and iron, too.

It's much healthier than frying because the heat encircles the meat and lets all of the fat drip off, away from the food so that you're not ingesting the added calories from the fat. What you end up with a lean cut of nutritious, juicy chicken to fuel your fat burning process.

The Ronco oven has a timer you can turn on that will let you cook for up to three hours and you can see how well it's doing by looking through the glass doors of the oven.

The spit that the meat goes on is a non stick variety, so clean up is a breeze. And there's a built in drip tray, along with a carving platter gloves for safety – to help your process go more smoothly.

The oven is small enough to fit on any counter. It's a little over fifteen inches high and almost eighteen inches wide. The oven is something many families love to use, instead of forking over much more to pick up a readymade rotisserie chicken at the grocery store (one of their most popular items for busy families, by the way).

Those who are adhering to a high protein, low carb diet to lose weight will be especially happy with the Ronco Rotisserie oven because it enables them to have a steady supply of flavorful meat for their meal plans.

Yum Yum Dishes

When you're trying to lose weight, one of the most common pieces of dieting advice you'll hear is to watch your portions. That's really hard, in a world where super-sized dishes have become the norm – no matter which meal (or snack) of the day you're eating.

There's an easy solution that makes portion control for your snacks a breeze – and we've all heard how eating six meals a day, with smaller portions, helps stave off weight gain and assists you in shedding pounds.

They're called **Yum Yum Dishes** (http://amzn.to/1J5Z9I9) and it's a set of four brightly colored, beautiful snack-sized bowls that dish up a 4-ounce serving of whatever it is you're eating. The best thing about the bowls is that it eliminates mindless eating – those moments where your hand is reaching in and out of the bag of chips until suddenly, the entire bag is gone!

These dishes are safe for the microwave and oven, and you can clean them easily by sticking them into the dishwasher for your next use. Consumers love how colorful they are. They come in a beautiful, bold blue, a bright cherry red, a cheerful sunshine yellow, and a yummy pistachio green shade.

If you want to store snacks in them, you can use the convenient snap on lids that come with them. That way you can prepare for mindful eating ahead of time and simply grab a bowl on your way out the door!

This isn't just a great weight loss tool for yourself. It's an incredible way to teach your kids mindful eating. There's a message hidden on the bottom of the bowl that says, "Over." When you've finished your snack, the bowl lets you (or your child) know.

A four-ounce portion isn't too big or too small. The Yum Yum Dishes are each three and a half inches in diameter and two inches tall. Perfect for fruit, nuts, or any variety of snack foods you want to use them for!

We all know that when we plan to just reach for a handful of Cheetos, it's very easy to keep reaching for one after another until you've not just eaten *one* serving, but three or four. With Yum Yum Dishes, you're given a handful – usually a single serving – and it's perfect for losing and maintaining weight loss.

These are not cheaply created dishes for toddlers. They're very well crafted with an artistic design – something adults will admire. They're not made of plastic, so you do still need to be careful in handling the bowls.

Most people welcome the dishes as an alternative to Ziploc baggies. It's especially helpful if you're using mindful eating and want to focus on the experience of mealtimes, using all of your senses.

Other Health and Fitness Books by This Author

If you would like to read more about Senior Health and Fitness, here is a list of the titles, CreateSpace links and descriptions:

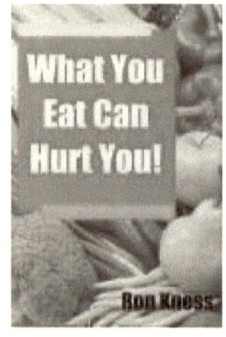

What You Eat Can Hurt You

https://www.createspace.com/4963196

Do you know that certain foods increase your risk for inflammation, disease and illness? It's true! And certain foods can help cure and heal you if you do get sick. Knowing which foods to eat and which ones to avoid empowers you to manage your own health.

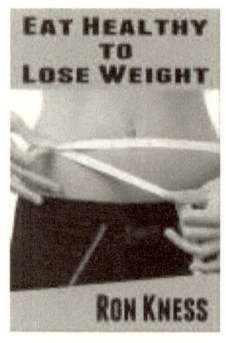

Eat Healthy to Lose Weight

https://www.createspace.com/4962939

As you read through our book, we show you which foods you should and should not be eating to reach your weight loss goal, along with discussing how to maintain your weight loss and stay within a few pounds of your goal weight. Banish the weight you keep gaining back each time by learning how to live a healthy lifestyle.

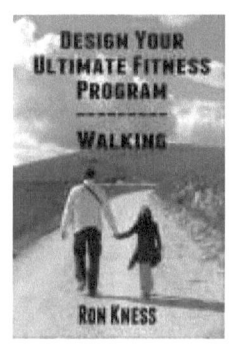

Design Your Ultimate Fitness Program - Walking

https://www.createspace.com/5252272

In my book Design Your Ultimate Fitness Program – Walking, we discuss the considerations that need to be made when designing a custom walking program, along with:

• Equipment needed
• Wearable technology you can use to track your walking
• And how to make walking more challenging

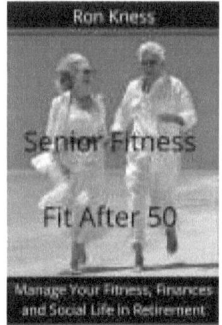

Senior Fitness – Fit After 50: Learn How to Manage Your Fitness, Finances and Social Life in Retirement

https://www.createspace.com/5474751

Inside you will discover answers to your most pressing questions:
• What do I need to know about downsizing my home?
• What are the best tips for staying healthy as you approach your 50's?
• When should I start planning for retirement?
• I am worried about being lonely once I retire, do others feel the same?
• Is it worthwhile to carry two homes during retirement?
And more…

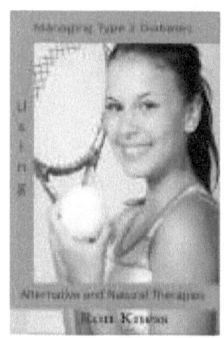

Managing Type 2 Diabetes Using Alternative And Natural Therapies

https://www.createspace.com/5401244

While Type 2 diabetes can be managed medically, there are many alternative natural and holistic methods of therapy and treatment that can further enhance quality of life and minimize the effects of this disease. In this book, I discuss 12 different types, including yoga, reflexology and acupuncture to name just three.

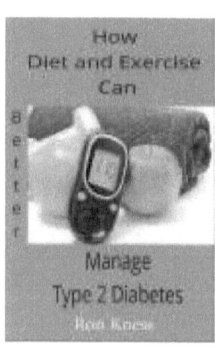

How Diet and Exercise Can Better Manage Type 2 Diabetes

https://www.createspace.com/5404845

Of the different types of diabetes, only Type 2 can be reversed. In my book How Diet and Exercise Can Better Manage Type 2 Diabetes, we reveal the three things you can do to best manage your disease, including:
• Diet
• Exercise
• Weight management

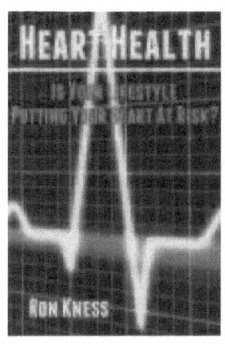

Heart Health: Is Your Lifestyle Putting Your Heart at Risk?

https://www.createspace.com/5464020

In my ebook Is Your Lifestyle Putting Your Heart At Risk? we discuss the six greatest risks to your heart and the lifestyle changes you can make to mitigate them.

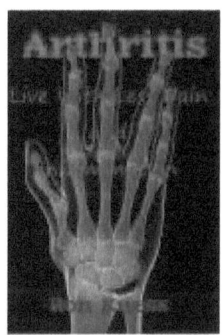

Arthritis – Live Wth Less Pain and Inflammation: Tips and Techniques You Can Use to Lessen the Pain and Inflammation

https://www.createspace.com/5457441

Discover Simple Tips & Information That Will Help Reduce The Painful Symptoms Of Arthritis!

You learn things like:
• Simple and effective information that will help you manage the pain and inflammation that comes along with arthritis, so that you can live an active, full life without debilitating pain.
• The different types of arthritis, their symptoms and how to alleviate their painful side effects.
• The pros and cons of over-the-counter arthritis medications, plus simple tips that will help you know how to choose the right supplements.
• Free, yet effective ways to get relief from arthritis pain and inflammation, so you don't have to suffer anymore.

The effects arthritis can have significant impact on your physical and mental well-being, but this books shows you how to overcome its painful symptoms and live life relatively pain free.

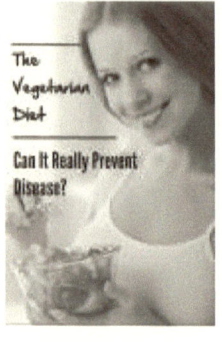

The Vegetarian Diet – Can It Really Prevent Disease?

https://www.createspace.com/5519874

Is a vegetarian diet right for you? Multiple studies have shown over and over that a vegetarian diet goes a long way in preventing certain chronic diseases, such as:

• Heart Disease
• Cancer
• Diverticulitis
• Type 2 Diabetes
• Hypertension
• Obesity
• Kidney Failure

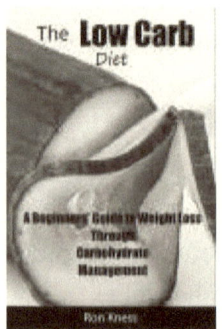

The Low Carb Diet: A Beginner's Guide to Weight Loss Through Carbohydrate Management

https://www.createspace.com/5416348

In my book "The Low-Carb Diet – A Beginners' Guide to Weight Loss Through Carbohydrate Management", I reveal a successful method of losing weight based in part on the amount and type of carbohydrates you consume.

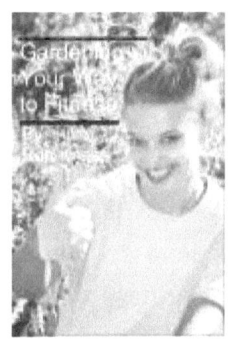

Gardening Your Way to Fitness: The Fun Way to Get Fit and Provide Beauty and Healthful Bounty for Your Family

https://www.createspace.com/5459564

The gym is a great place to stay fit during the colder seasons, but once the temperature turns warmer you want to spend more time outside. Plus, you'll have the benefit of fresh wholesome produce to enjoy by growing vegetables in your backyard garden.

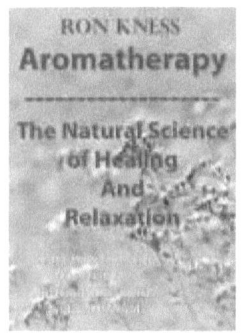

Aromatherapy - The Science of Healing and Relaxation: Learn How Essential Oils Elicit The Relaxation Response And Alter Mood

https://www.createspace.com/5714434

In my book Aromatherapy – The Science of Healing and Relaxation, we reveal the natural holistics methods you can use to heal the body from certain medical issues and to relive stress through relaxation. In particular we talk about:
• Aromatherapy - what it is and how it works
• Essential Oils – how the effects of certain aromas differs from others
• Recipes – how to make your own essential oil combinations

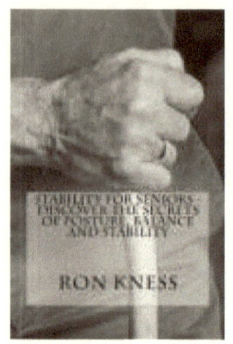

Stability for Seniors: Discover the Secrets of Posture, Balance and Stability

https://www.createspace.com/6096479

Many people sacrifice their health in pursuit of their career. They are so busy making a living that they neglect to make a life. The excuse that they do not have time to exercise is tossed about so frequently that they end up letting their health and fitness slide.

If you are not regularly active, you will have muscular atrophy over time. Your flexibility will decrease. Your core strength will diminish. As time progresses, you will be less limber and more rigid.

This is exactly how people age poorly. It's a process that has snowballed over time.

Only with regular exercise and a healthy diet can you have a body that is fit and has the ability to almost reverse aging.

If you have neglected your health for years and life seems to be a chore now because you can't get around without assistance, do not feel dejected.

You can remedy the situation. You can restore the strength, balance and stamina that you have lost. It is never too late to become what you might have been.

This guide will show you exactly what you need to do to restore your balance, strengthen your core and give you the ability to live life to its fullest. Read how …

About the Author

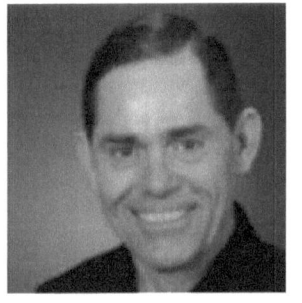

I grew up in Central Minnesota, where my parents own and operated a fishing resort. Once out of high school I tried a couple of semesters of college, only to quit halfway through the Spring term; I decided at that time that college wasn't for me.

Then I decided to follow my father's previous occupation as an auto mechanic. I graduated from a two-year of vocational training course and worked as a mechanic. While in vocational training, I decided to join the National Guard where I eventually ended up working full-time for 32 years.

So how does all of this relate to writing? In one of my leadership schools, the instructor, who was an English teacher at a juvenile detention center, presented writing to me in a whole new way - a way that started to develop my interest in working with words.

Fast forward about 40 years and I now have over 50 books listed on Amazon for Kindle and CreateSpace.